Surviving Morning Sickness

A Personal Journey of Triumph and Hope by a Hyperemesis Gravidarum Warrior

Isabella White

Copyright © 2023 by Isabella White.

The publisher reserves all rights. Without prior written permission, no part of this publication may be reproduced, distributed, or transmitted in any form or by any means, including photocopying, recording, or other electronic or mechanical methods. Under copyright law, limited quotations may be used for non-commercial purposes and critical reviews.

***Disclaimer:** The information in this book is based on the author's research, opinions, and experiences. It is not intended to replace professional medical advice or treatment. The reader should regularly consult a physician for any health issues and always seek the advice of a physician before modifying diet, supplement, or exercise regimens. The author and publisher shall have neither liability nor responsibility to any person or entity concerning any loss or damage related to the information contained in this book. The information provided is general and may not apply to every individual. Any reliance on the information contained herein is solely at the reader's risk.*

Table of Contents

Introduction

I was overjoyed when I learned I was pregnant with my daughter. My husband and I had been trying to conceive for nearly a year and eagerly anticipated this new chapter of our lives together. However, that excitement soon turned into misery once the nausea and vomiting kicked in around week 6 of my pregnancy.

At first, I assumed it was normal morning sickness and tried to push through it. I could barely keep anything down, not even water, but people kept telling me it would pass. By week 9, I had lost nearly 12 pounds and was growing severely dehydrated. That is when I was finally diagnosed with hyperemesis gravidarum.

What followed was the most challenging nine months I have ever faced. The nausea and vomiting were relentless, causing me to lose an unhealthy amount of weight and landing me in the hospital for IV fluids every few weeks. I felt completely debilitated and depressed. Taking care of my toddler son became impossible. I had to take an extended leave from my job. I became isolated from friends and family because I was too ill to leave the house.

Everyday tasks like cooking, cleaning, and showering were huge hurdles due to my extreme fatigue and weakness. My husband had to take over everything while still working to support us financially. We incurred substantial medical bills from frequent hospital visits and medications. Our relationship was strained under the stress.

I honestly did not know how I would survive those nine months or how I could cope with hyperemesis again if we decided to expand our family in the future. It took every ounce of strength to make it through each day. With the help of my doctors, my husband's support, and sheer determination, I finally made it to delivery day.

Though my case was severe, I know many women suffer even more severely for longer durations. Living through hyperemesis made me realize the importance of awareness, proper medical treatment, emotional support, and having an empathetic healthcare team. My mission now is to use my experience to help other hyperemesis gravidarum warriors in their journey and improve care for this debilitating pregnancy complication. If I can help even one woman feel less alone on this difficult road, it makes my battle worthwhile.

Definition of Hyperemesis Gravidarum

Hyperemesis gravidarum is a condition characterized by severe and persistent nausea and vomiting during pregnancy. While nausea and vomiting are common during the first trimester of pregnancy, hyperemesis gravidarum is much more extreme, resulting in dehydration, nutritional deficiencies, and weight loss.

The main distinguishing factor of hyperemesis gravidarum is the severity and duration of symptoms. Nausea and vomiting occur on an almost constant basis, making it difficult or impossible to keep down food and liquids. This leads to electrolyte imbalances and often requires hospitalization for hydration and nutrition via IV fluids and medications.

Whereas regular morning sickness symptoms peak around week 9 of pregnancy and subside by week 16, hyperemesis gravidarum persists well into the second trimester and sometimes lasts the entire pregnancy. Nausea and vomiting are so severe that women are unable to care for themselves and carry out daily activities.

Although the precise causes of hyperemesis gravidarum are unknown, genetics and hormonal changes are considered to be involved. Levels of the pregnancy hormone hCG are often higher in women with hyperemesis. The condition also tends to run in families. Additional risk factors include maternal age, multiple pregnancies, obesity, trophoblastic disease, and hydatidiform mole.

Some key facts about hyperemesis gravidarum:

- It usually begins before the ninth week of pregnancy, but symptoms can start at 4–5 weeks.
- Up to 3–5% of pregnant women experience hyperemesis gravidarum.
- It involves vomiting several times a day and an inability to keep down food or liquids.
- It can lead to dehydration, electrolyte imbalance, malnutrition, and weight loss.
- It requires medical treatment such as IV fluids, vitamin supplements, and anti-nausea medications.
- Symptoms usually improve by week 16 but may last throughout the pregnancy.
- It can recur in subsequent pregnancies.

The debilitating symptoms of hyperemesis gravidarum can take a serious physical and emotional toll on expectant mothers. Unlike regular morning sickness, hyperemesis prevents women from being able to care for themselves and function normally on a day-to-day basis. Proper treatment and support are crucial.

Hyperemesis gravidarum affects approximately 1–2% of pregnancies, though prevalence rates may vary slightly by country and population. This means it impacts tens of thousands of women annually in the United States alone. The condition is more commonly seen in women pregnant with their first child, in teenage pregnancies, and in multiple gestations like twins or triplets.

Despite how severely it impacts those who suffer from it, hyperemesis gravidarum often goes minimized or undiagnosed. Many women are told they need to "power through" their symptoms because they are an extreme form of the common morning sickness. This leads to prolonged suffering and poor pregnancy outcomes.

When left improperly managed, hyperemesis gravidarum can have significant adverse effects on maternal and fetal health as well as overall pregnancy.

1. **Dehydration, malnourishment, and weight loss in mothers.** Persistent vomiting and the inability to keep down nutrients can cause severe weight loss and vitamin and mineral deficiencies. Dehydration alters the electrolyte balance.

2. **Hospitalization.** Around 60% of women with hyperemesis require hospitalization for IV fluids and nutrition. The average hospital stay is three days, which can take 7–10 days.

3. **Emotional distress.** Coping with unrelenting nausea or vomiting leads to anxiety, depression, and difficulty bonding.

4. **Pregnancy complications.** Research links hyperemesis to an increased risk of low birth weight, preterm delivery, and small for gestational-age babies.

5. **Recurrence in subsequent pregnancies.** Up to 80% of sufferers experience hyperemesis again in later pregnancies. This can discourage family planning.

6. **Loss of time or activities.** The condition prevents women from working, caring for family, attending events or outings, and engaging in everyday activities.

7. **Healthcare costs.** Hospitalizations and additional care result in an estimated $200 million annually in increased healthcare spending.

With proper medical treatment and emotional support, many of the effects of hyperemesis can be reduced or managed. The key is for healthcare providers to recognize the severity of this condition early so women can get the help they need. Effective treatment can help mitigate risks and preserve quality of life, even in severe cases.

Chapter 1

Understanding Hyperemesis Gravidarum

The Causes and Medical Background

Hyperemesis gravidarum has been recognized as a distinct medical condition for over a century. However, its exact causes are still not entirely understood. Research points to a complex interaction of physiological, genetic, and environmental factors that trigger this extreme nausea and vomiting during pregnancy.

From a physiological standpoint, the high levels of hCG and estrogens that support pregnancy appear to play a primary role. These hormones steadily rise during the first trimester, which correlates with when hyperemesis symptoms start for most women. The rapidly shifting hormonal milieu disrupts the normal functioning of the gastrointestinal tract and central nervous system.

Abnormalities in other pregnancy-related hormones like thyroxine and prolactin may also contribute. Additionally, Helicobacter pylori infection and abnormalities in liver function are associated with more severe hyperemesis gravidarum.

Genetics is another strong predictor. Women whose mothers suffered from hyperemesis gravidarum have an over 3-fold increased risk of developing it themselves. Specific gene mutations related to retinoid and steroid hormone metabolism have been implicated.

Environmental influences may provide the tipping point for genetically susceptible women. Stress and anxiety during pregnancy can aggravate symptoms. Exposure to nausea or vomiting triggers like certain smells or foods also plays a role for some women.

Experts believe that hyperemesis gravidarum occurs in a subset of pregnant women due to a combination of factors, including individual genetic and environmental vulnerabilities, as well as the body's natural response to the rise in pregnancy hormones.

While the exact mechanisms are still being unraveled, it is clear that:

- Hormone changes alone do not explain the severity of HG. Most women have elevated hCG, but far fewer develop HG.
- Not all cases of HG can be explained by changes in other hormone levels.
- Genetics underlie susceptibility but do not fully predict outcomes.
- Environmental factors alone do not trigger HG but can exacerbate underlying genetic risk.

Ongoing research aims to understand these variables better and develop prognostic tests to identify at-risk women. Advancing knowledge of the pathogenesis can also open doors for more targeted, effective treatments.

Differentiating Normal Morning Sickness from Hyperemesis Gravidarum

Nausea and vomiting affect up to 80% of expectant mothers during early pregnancy. Commonly referred to as morning sickness, these symptoms typically begin around week 6, peak around week 9, and resolve by weeks 16–18. While unpleasant, morning sickness is generally manageable for most women. Hyperemesis gravidarum, on the other hand, is debilitating and life-altering.

The key differences between morning sickness and hyperemesis gravidarum include:

1. **Severity of nausea or vomiting:** Morning sickness causes mild to moderate nausea and vomiting that comes and goes. Hyperemesis leads to constant, severe vomiting up to over ten times a day.

2. **Ability to keep down food and liquids:** With morning sickness, women can generally keep some nutrients and fluids. Sufferers of hyperemesis are often unable to keep anything down for extended periods.

3. **Timing and duration:** Morning sickness peaks around nine weeks and improves by week 16. Hyperemesis persists well into the 2nd and sometimes the entire third trimester.

4. **Impact on daily life:** Regular morning sickness allows continuation of most normal activities like

work, social events, family care, exercise, etc. Hyperemesis prevents normal function.

5. **Weight loss:** Some minor weight loss can occur with morning sickness. Hyperemesis frequently leads to over 5% body weight loss from severe dehydration and malnutrition.

6. **Need for treatment:** Lifestyle changes usually manage morning sickness. Hyperemesis requires IV fluids and nutrition, hospitalization, and medication.

7. **Recurrence risk:** Morning sickness differs with each pregnancy. Hyperemesis recurs around 80% of the time with subsequent pregnancies.

8. **Emotional toll:** Morning sickness can cause some stress and frustration. Hyperemesis takes a heavy psychological toll and often leads to depression or anxiety.

The severity of symptoms, level of impairment, and risk to maternal and fetal health help distinguish hyperemesis gravidarum from even the worst regular cases of morning sickness. Seeking prompt medical treatment is crucial to preventing complications. With proper care, women can achieve healthier pregnancies.

The Impact on Maternal and Fetal Health

Hyperemesis gravidarum can significantly impact both maternal and fetal health if left improperly managed. Understanding these risks is key to proper treatment and monitoring during pregnancy.

For the mother, the most immediate threat is dehydration and nutritional deficiencies from persistent vomiting and an inability to keep down food or liquids. This leads to electrolyte imbalances, vitamin and mineral depletion, and dangerous levels of ketones in the blood from the breakdown of fat for energy.

Low carbohydrate intake and dehydration also diminish the fetus's essential volume and nutrient delivery. Nutrient deficiencies may cause headaches, muscle wasting, weakness, anemia, and altered mental status.

Secondary risks arise from these primary complications. Severe dehydration and electrolyte derangements can progress to kidney failure or arrhythmias. Skeletal and neurological issues can develop from vitamin or mineral depletion over time.

The woman's immune function may also become impaired, predisposing her to infections. Anxiety and depression are common emotional side effects as well.

Maternal malnutrition and volume depletion for the developing fetus reduce the delivery of oxygen and nutrients essential for growth and organ development. Babies of mothers with severe hyperemesis are at higher risk of:

- Intrauterine growth restriction and low birth weight
- Small size for gestational age
- Preterm delivery
- Congenital disabilities like neural tube defects and cleft lip/palate.

The likelihood of these outcomes appears to be directly related to the severity and duration of maternal symptoms and the timing of weight loss. Catching and properly managing hyperemesis early on can help mitigate many of these complications.

Most women can achieve significantly improved nutrition and hydration status with IV fluid and nutrition, vitamin supplementation, anti-emetic medications, and electrolyte monitoring. This supports better fetal development.

Close monitoring of fetal growth parameters and anatomy ultrasounds is also essential for the early detection of any fetal abnormalities. Prompt treatment coupled with vigilant monitoring allows the majority of hyperemesis pregnancies to still result in positive outcomes for both mother and baby.

Chapter 2

Recognizing the Signs and Symptoms

Early Indicators of Hyperemesis Gravidarum

During the first several weeks of pregnancy, it can be difficult to differentiate normal morning sickness from more severe nausea that might signal hyperemesis gravidarum. However, recognizing the early signs and symptoms can help ensure prompt treatment and better pregnancy outcomes.

Key red flags in the first trimester include:

1. **Intractable nausea:** Nausea that persists throughout the day and is not relieved by changes in

activity, diet, or environment. It feels constant and unavoidable.

2. **Vomiting frequently:** Vomiting several times daily, sometimes for hours at a time. This prevents keeping down any food or liquids.

3. **Excessive salivation:** Continuously overproducing saliva that fills the mouth and triggers vomiting episodes. This is when you have to swallow a lot of spittle.

4. **Weight loss:** Losing 5% or more of pre-pregnancy body weight by week 12 due to constant vomiting and diarrhea.

5. **Ketosis:** Developing high ketone levels in the urine from the body, breaking down fat for fuel instead of glucose. This upsets the electrolyte balance.

6. **Dehydration:** Dry mouth or lips; dark or decreased urination; racing heart rate; dizziness upon standing. Headaches and muscle cramps may also occur.

7. **Inability to complete daily tasks:** Simple activities like getting dressed, fixing meals, or going to work become impossible due to fatigue and weakness.

Women exhibiting these signs within the first trimester, especially by week 9, should be evaluated for hyperemesis gravidarum. The frequency and duration of symptoms also matter; occasionally, vomiting versus keeping nothing down all day points to HG.

Prompt initiation of IV fluids, anti-nausea medications, vitamin supplements, and a care plan for monitoring and treating symptoms can help stabilize the mother and protect the pregnancy. Catching HG early and administering appropriate treatment is crucial.

Severity Levels and When to Seek Medical Help

Hyperemesis gravidarum occurs along a spectrum of severity. Recognizing when symptoms have progressed from mild to moderate to severe helps guide the appropriate medical evaluation and treatment timing.

Mild HG involves nausea or vomiting multiple times per day that impairs regular function but responds partially to lifestyle changes. Weight loss of up to 5% of pre-pregnancy body weight may occur. This level usually warrants anti-nausea medication and regular monitoring by a doctor.

Regular vomiting and nausea that do not go away with rest or medicine are signs of moderate HG. Weight loss of 5–10% of pre-pregnancy weight is common. The woman is unable to maintain adequate nutrition and hydration orally.

Outpatient IV fluid treatment is often needed a few times a week, along with other anti-nausea and nutritional interventions.

Severe HG involves debilitating symptoms that prevent any oral intake, resulting in dehydration, significant electrolyte imbalances, and over 10% body weight loss. Hospitalization for IV nutrition, hydration, and medications becomes essential to stabilize the woman's health and support the pregnancy.

Key indicators of when to seek urgent medical evaluation and treatment include:

- Inability to retain any food or liquids by mouth for over 24 hours
- Weight loss exceeding 5% of pre-pregnancy weight
- Dark urine or urinating less than 2-3 times per day (signs of dehydration)
- Lightheadedness, racing heart rate, or fainting upon standing
- Presence of ketones in urine (a sign of starvation metabolism)
- Dry mouth, eyes, or skin that lacks normal elasticity
- Persistent headache, muscle cramps, or other symptoms of electrolyte imbalance

- Feeling depressed, hopeless, or unable to function normally

Seeking prompt medical care for escalating symptoms can curb complications and relieve suffering. With the right treatment team, even women with severe HG can go on to have healthy pregnancies and babies. Remaining in denial or delaying treatment puts both mother and child at greater risk. Please do not assume it is normal morning sickness; seek help early.

Common Misconceptions about Morning Sickness

There are many myths and misconceptions about morning sickness that lead women and even some healthcare providers to minimize or overlook the signs of hyperemesis gravidarum. Dispelling these pregnancy-related falsehoods is crucial for proper diagnosis and treatment.

Common morning sickness myths include:

1. **It only occurs in the morning.** Nausea can strike at any time of day or night with regular morning sickness and hyperemesis gravidarum. The "morning" term is a misnomer.

2. **It is a sign of a healthy pregnancy.** While mild nausea may signal hormonal changes that support fetal growth, severe vomiting, and weight loss are never normal or healthy.

3. **It is always resolved by the second trimester.** Most regular morning sickness resolves by week 16, but hyperemesis persists well beyond that for many women.

4. **It is just an exaggeration of normal queasiness.** HG is a real, serious maternal-fetal health disorder, not just an amplified normal symptom.

5. **Eating crackers is the first thing that can prevent it.** There is no known way to prevent hyperemesis gravidarum, though eating before getting up may help with minor morning nausea.

6. **Women need to power through it.** Attempting to ignore hyperemesis can have dire consequences, including fetal and maternal malnutrition.

7. **It is psychological or attention-seeking.** While anxiety may worsen queasiness, HG has physiological causes, not mental health roots.

8. **Natural remedies are sufficient.** HG requires medical treatment, not just ginger tea, sea bands, vitamin B6, or positive thinking.

9. **Bed rest cures it.** Rest may help relieve general pregnancy discomfort, but it does not resolve HG's severe vomiting and dehydration.

Dispelling these common myths among patients and healthcare teams is imperative to speed up diagnosis and treatment. Left unchecked, the misconception that hyperemesis gravidarum is just an exaggerated form of normal morning sickness causes needless suffering and puts mother and child at risk. Education and advocacy are key to improving care.

Chapter 3

Coping Strategies for Navigating Daily Challenges

Dietary Modifications and Nutritional Tips

Finding ways to adapt one's diet is an important part of coping with hyperemesis gravidarum. While no food can cure HG, certain approaches may help sufferers get increased nutrition and hydration when vomiting permits.

Top tips include:

1. **Eat small, frequent meals.** 5–6 mini-meals spaced regularly throughout the day are easier to tolerate than large meals.

2. **Focus on well-tolerated foods.** Stick to bland, easy-to-digest foods that seem to "stay down" better, like bananas, rice, toast, and crackers. Avoid spicy, fatty, or pungent triggers.

3. **Try cold or room-temperature foods.** Hot foods can exacerbate nausea with their strong smells. Cooler foods may be better tolerated.

4. **Eat protein-rich snacks.** Getting adequate protein is crucial when intake is limited. Try nuts, Greek yogurt, cheese, or peanut butter.

5. **Intersperse fluids between bites.** Sip water, herbal tea, broth, or diluted juices constantly with meals. Fluids make it hard to get down alone when nauseated.

6. **Eat before getting out of bed.** Start with dry foods like crackers before moving to avoid triggering nausea.

7. **Stay upright after eating.** Remain vertical for at least 30 minutes post-meals to aid digestion and minimize regurgitation.

8. **Rinse your taste buds between bites.** Sour flavors can refresh the palate. Suck on lemon drops, frozen mango, or tart candies between nibbles.

9. **Use ginger.** Ginger tea, popsicles, and candies may help calm nausea without medication.

10. **Get nutrients from enriched drinks.** Protein shakes, smoothies with spinach or avocado, and electrolyte solutions provide an easier absorption route.

11. **Take vitamin supplements.** Prenatal vitamins and supplements for deficiencies identified by bloodwork can help fill nutritional gaps.

The key is to eat whatever is tolerable at that moment and continue trying different tricks to get calories and hydration in any way possible. Remaining flexible and monitoring weight and nutritional status for more intensive interventions as needed are key.

Hydration Techniques for Managing Severe Nausea

Dehydration from persistent vomiting is a major hazard of hyperemesis gravidarum. Finding ways to maintain hydration is crucial for the health of both the mother and the developing baby. Helpful techniques include:

1. **Take small, frequent sips.** Drink just a tablespoon or two of fluid every 5–10 minutes rather than large amounts. This is easier to tolerate and absorb.

2. **Try oral rehydration solutions.** Drinks like Pedialyte contain optimal sodium and glucose levels to aid absorption.

3. **Alternate between cold and room temperature.** Some women find icy drinks easier, while others prefer tepid fluids. Have both on hand.

4. **Set reminder alarms.** Schedule alerts on your phone to remind you to take in more fluid throughout the day.

5. **Make electrolyte popsicles.** Freeze electrolyte drinks or coconut water into nourishing pops to help you stay hydrated.

6. **Add flavor enhancers.** A squeeze of lemon, fruit puree, or a hint of ginger can make plain water more palatable.

7. **Use chamomile or mint tea.** Herbal teas can provide soothing aromas and needed fluids.

8. **Keep the water visible.** Have water bottles, cups, or straws available on your nightstand, couch, or office to prompt more intake.

9. **Set goals for urine color.** Aim for very pale yellow urine to ensure adequate hydration.

10. **Monitor your weight.** Sudden drops signal fluid loss and the need for more aggressive IV hydration measures.

11. **Try IV hydration at home.** IV clinics can provide outpatient infusions a few times a week to keep you from getting severely dehydrated.

12. **Use anti-nausea medication.** Getting vomiting under better control can help fluid intake indirectly.

The key is experimenting to find a variety of tolerable hydration sources. Hospitalization for IV fluid and nutrition may still be needed periodically, but implementing these techniques can help reduce the frequency of that more intensive intervention.

Rest and Self-care Practices

Hyperemesis gravidarum can be physically and emotionally exhausting. Making rest and self-care a priority is vital to coping with the condition. Useful strategies include:

1. **Sleep and nap frequently.** The severe nausea and vomiting are extremely frustrating. Allow your body to rest when needed.

2. **Create a soothing sleep environment.** Eye masks, earplugs, comfortable pillows, and bedding can all promote better-quality sleep.

3. **Ask for help.** Refrain from trying to push through with housework or caregiving. Have family assist with chores or errands.

4. **Set up a sick room.** Have a space with supplies and distractions to minimize movement on bad days.

5. **Stay hydrated.** Dehydration exacerbates fatigue and headaches. Keep electrolyte drinks and popsicles on hand.

6. **Use Sea-Bands:** These acupressure wristbands may help reduce nausea for some women.

7. **Take warm baths.** Warm water can be soothing physically and psychologically. Add Epsom salts to replenish magnesium.

8. **Apply peppermint oil.** Its cooling aromatherapy effect may reduce nausea. Dilute before applying to the wrists or temples.

9. **Listen to guided meditation.** Soothing apps can aid relaxation when nausea disrupts sleep.

10. **Join a support group.** Connecting with other women battling HG can ease isolation and fear.

11. **Consider therapy.** A therapist provides emotional support and coping skills.
12. **Be kind to yourself.** This is not your fault. Focus on doing whatever you can manage each day.
13. **Recruit childcare help.** Do not try to care for other kids alone. Ask your family to pitch in.
14. **Communicate with your employer.** Discuss flex scheduling or working from home to accommodate your condition.

Remember, perfection is not the goal—merely survival. Rest, hydrate, take medications, and do not feel guilty about needing extra help. ***This will pass.***

Chapter 4

Medical Interventions and Treatments

Overview of Available Medications

While no single medication can cure hyperemesis gravidarum, there are several pharmaceutical options available to help control symptoms. Anti-nausea and acid-reducing medications are the mainstays of treatment.

Types of medications used include:

1. **Antihistamines:** Antivert, Diclegis, and Bonjesta contain doxylamine, an antihistamine with anticholinergic and anti-nausea effects. These are considered safe for pregnancy.

2. **Anticholinergics:** Scopolamine patches or oral meds like Dramamine have anticholinergic properties to reduce nausea and vomiting. Not all are pregnancy-approved.

3. **Dopamine antagonists:** Reglan, Phenergan, and Compazine block dopamine receptors to reduce nausea. The risk of dystonic reactions exists.

4. **5-HT3 receptor antagonists:** Zofran and ondansetron block serotonin receptors involved in nausea. One of the most commonly used HG medications.

5. **Benzodiazepines:** Anti-anxiety medications like Xanax may treat associated depression or anxiety, exacerbating nausea.

6. **Corticosteroids:** Steroids help reduce inflammation implicated in severe nausea and vomiting. Used only in refractory cases given risks.

7. **Proton pump inhibitors:** (PPIs) like Prilosec or Protonix suppress gastric acid secretion, which can worsen symptoms.

Typically, patients start with safer options like antihistamines, anticholinergics, and serotonin receptor blockers. If nausea remains uncontrolled, providers may try adding benzodiazepines, dopamine antagonists, or corticosteroids with caution.

Finding the right medication or combination takes some trial and error. The goal is to use the least invasive options at the lowest effective doses to control vomiting and allow hydration and nutrition. Close monitoring of the baby is also needed to ensure proper development. With an experienced maternal-fetal medicine team, HG medication regimens can be optimized for the health of both mother and child.

The Potential Risks and Benefits

When considering medications to treat hyperemesis gravidarum, weighing the potential risks against the benefits to both the mother and the developing baby is important.

For the benefits, anti-nausea and anti-vomiting medications provide the primary advantage of reducing or controlling the constant nausea and vomiting, allowing better nutrition and hydration. This can:

- Prevent hospitalization from severe dehydration or starvation.
- Enable weight stabilization and modest weight gain.

- Resolve vitamin and mineral deficiencies.
- Reduce ketonuria and associated electrolyte derangements.
- Improve emotional health by alleviating symptoms.

Controlling symptoms also lowers the risk of serious maternal complications like kidney injury, arrhythmias, and nutrient deficiencies, as well as poor fetal outcomes like growth restriction, congenital disabilities, and preterm birth.

However, medications do carry risks, including:

- Potential fetal exposure and placental transfer of chemicals.
- Unknown long-term neurodevelopmental effects on the baby.
- Adverse maternal reactions like headaches, constipation, and drowsiness.
- Safety concerns with certain medication classes in pregnancy.
- Dosing challenges due to pharmacokinetic changes in pregnancy.

Generally, the benefits of treating severe nausea and vomiting outweigh the risks of untreated HG. However, providers must select medications carefully based on trimester, avoid polypharmacy when possible, use the minimum effective dose, and monitor fetal development closely.

By working closely with a high-risk maternal-fetal medicine specialist and sticking to the safest medications at the lowest doses, most women with HG can experience significant symptom improvement without major fetal risks. However, medications alone are not a cure-all; nutritional support, IV fluids, and nutrients are also key. An integrated plan customized for the patient offers the best outcome for mom and baby.

Alternative Therapies and Their Efficacy

In addition to medications, some women with hyperemesis gravidarum turn to alternative or complementary therapies in hopes of relieving their constant nausea and vomiting.

Common options include:

1. **Acupuncture:** This involves placing thin needles at specific points on the body to restore proper energy flow. Small studies show some benefits for nausea reduction.

2. **Ginger:** Available as ginger ale, teas, candies, or capsules. It may help with mild nausea but lacks strong evidence for efficacy in severe HG.

3. **Peppermint:** This can be taken as a tea, essential oil, or aromatherapy. It may reduce nausea mildly, but data is limited.

4. **Probiotics:** These healthy gut bacteria supplements could improve GI issues linked to HG, but supporting research is sparse.

5. **Pyridoxine (vitamin B6):** This is often combined with doxylamine in the Diclegis formulation, showing HG efficacy. Alone, B6 has yet to prove effective.

6. **Thiamine (vitamin B1):** Thought to help correct nutritional deficiencies aggravating nausea but not rigorously studied for HG treatment.

7. **Acupressure:** Applying pressure to the inner wrist area with bracelets or massage may activate pathways to decrease nausea. Limited data exists.

8. **Cannabinoids:** Marijuana derivatives like CBD oils are considered possibly effective against severe nausea. However, data on pregnancy is scarce.

9. **Homeopathy:** Using highly dilute natural preparations to stimulate healing. No high-quality studies support homeopathy for HG treatment.

While many women report success with some of these alternatives, there is a lack of large, rigorous studies demonstrating a significant impact on HG symptoms specifically. They likely pose little harm and may be worth trying, but they should not replace standard medical treatment.

If choosing alternatives, it is essential to consult doctors to ensure safety during pregnancy and avoid interactions with prescribed medications. Most providers recommend approaches like acupuncture and ginger as complements, not wholesale alternatives, to necessary IV fluids, vitamin supplementation, and pharmaceutical anti-nausea medications. A coordinated plan combining evidence-based conventional treatments with certain complementary therapies may offer optimal relief for both mother and baby.

Chapter 5

Emotional Toll and Support Systems

Impact on Mental Health

In addition to the grueling physical symptoms, hyperemesis gravidarum often takes a heavy emotional toll. The unrelenting nausea, vomiting, and fatigue can lead to feelings of depression, anxiety, isolation, and hopelessness in expectant mothers. Up to 50% of women with HG experience clinical depression. Causes are multifactorial, including:

- Frustration and demoralization from constant vomiting and an inability to function normally

- Embarrassment about vomiting constantly in public or at social or work events
- Guilt over being unable to care for family members or perform daily responsibilities
- Fear over the health risks to the baby from malnutrition and dehydration
- Disappointment and resentment over the inability to enjoy the pregnancy
- Anger toward healthcare providers who downplay symptoms as normal
- Loneliness and disconnect from friends or family who does not understand the severity
- The loss of personal joy and excitement that often accompanies pregnancy
- Lack of control over one's body and life circumstances
- Exhaustion from an inability to get normal sleep and nutrition

HG's physical toll makes it difficult to muster coping skills and perspective. Depression exacerbates nausea, while malnutrition depletes serotonin, worsening the mood. It becomes a vicious cycle.

Seeking mental health support is as critical as medical care. Psychotherapy, support groups, family counseling, and even antidepressants can help women cope emotionally. Preventing isolation and promoting hope are imperatives.

With compassionate emotional support and proper treatment, the depression and anxiety accompanying HG often resolve postpartum. Nevertheless, active management of the mental health impact of HG is crucial; treatment cannot just focus on the physical. Maternal-fetal medicine teams must address psychological well-being to optimize outcomes.

Building a Support Network

Battling hyperemesis gravidarum can feel extremely isolating. Establishing a strong support network is vital to helping mothers physically and emotionally cope. Key components of a support system include:

1. **Family Support:** Spouses, parents, and immediate family members need to be educated about HG's severity to provide better emotional and physical support. Couples counseling helps process relationship strain.

2. **Friends:** Reach out to close friends, especially those who have experienced pregnancy. Their visits, texts, and encouragement counter isolation. Choose who you spend your limited energy on carefully.

3. **Workplace:** Communicate challenges to employers and negotiate accommodations like telecommuting or flex schedules. Understand your rights under pregnancy and disability laws.

4. **Childcare:** Recruit family members to help care for other kids when HG has you bedridden. Prioritize your rest and health.

5. **Household help:** Ask loved ones to pitch in with chores, errands, shopping, and hygiene that become difficult. Accept offers of meal help.

6. **Medical team:** Find an ob-gynecologist and perinatologist well-versed in HG who provides compassionate, proactive care. Dietitians can help tailor nutritional advice.

7. **Mental health support:** Seek out a therapist to help develop coping skills and process complex emotions. Join an HG support group.

8. **Online forums:** Connect with fellow HG moms through sites like HELLP and Hyperemesis Education and Research to find solidarity.

9. **Alternative practitioners:** Some find relief in seeking acupuncture, massage, or chiropractic care for symptom management. Verify safety.

10. **Finances:** Get information on insurance coverage, disability aid, and prescription financial assistance to ease monetary stress.

Having people to lean on for emotional and logistical support makes coping with HG's daily challenges feasible. Letting go of embarrassment, pride, and isolation is key. You do not have to power through this alone. ***Build your village.***

Professional Counseling and Mental Wellness Strategies

In addition to support from loved ones, professional mental health guidance can be invaluable in navigating the emotional toll of hyperemesis gravidarum. Counseling provides coping skills and perspective.

Seeking a perinatal psychiatrist or therapist experienced in high-risk pregnancies offers specialized expertise. Many focus on:

- Processing grief over the loss of a normal pregnancy experience

- Managing fears about health complications for mom and baby,
- Overcoming resentment toward caregivers or family, not understanding the severity,
- Coping with identity shifts and loss of independence or control,
- Combating social isolation and building a compassionate support network
- Fostering self-kindness and eliminating unfounded guilt
- Enhancing relationship communication skills as couples navigate challenges
- Reducing anxieties about having to parent young children while severely ill
- Exploring existential struggles unique to those battling chronic illness

In addition to taking therapy approaches, mental wellness strategies can include:

- Keeping a gratitude journal to shift focus from suffering to blessings
- Practicing mindfulness and grounding techniques to manage nausea and anxiety

- Framing each day as a success rather than fixating on failures to function
- Eliminating negative self-talk and replacing it with encouragement
- Pursuing creative arts like painting or writing to nourish the spirit
- Capturing hopeful affirmations on paper to post around the home
- Limiting time on social media that elicits envy or negative comparisons
- Joining HG online forums to find community and know *"you are not alone."*

Remember, battling this level of nausea requires gentleness with oneself. Counseling and self-care aid in coping, so HG does not need to overshadow all joy during pregnancy. ***You will get through this.***

Chapter 6

Balancing Work and Personal Life

Communicating with Employers and Colleagues

Hyperemesis gravidarum can significantly impact a woman's ability to maintain her normal work duties and schedule. Open, understanding communication with employers and colleagues makes balancing work and hyperemesis more feasible. Key tips for effectively communicating HG at work include:

1. **Educating them about HG**. Explain that it is an extreme form of morning sickness requiring

medical intervention, not just standard pregnancy nausea. Share resources explaining its seriousness.

2. **Be honest about your limitations.** Do not downplay your symptoms. Explain specifically what tasks or schedules are problematic and why.

3. **Suggest realistic accommodations.** Propose solutions like shifting hours, flex scheduling, working from home, or temporary reassignment.

4. **Enlist your doctor's input.** Have your provider contact them to verify that it is a legitimate medical condition requiring accommodation.

5. **Refer to company policies.** Check the employee handbook or disability/leave policies that may support your requested accommodations.

6. **Know your legal rights.** Be familiar with the Pregnancy, Disability, and Leave Acts and the Americans with Disabilities Act in case advocacy is needed.

7. **Express your willingness to collaborate.** Make it clear that you wish to work cooperatively toward a solution, not just quit working.

8. **Share the good news along with the challenges.** Balance the discussion of HG's struggles with positive updates on your pregnancy.

9. **Keep communication open.** Provide ongoing updates so they understand it is a persistent issue requiring long-term flexibility.

10. **Convey gratitude for understanding.** Thank colleagues who pitch in or offer emotional support during the process.

Most employers and coworkers will express empathy and willingness to solve problems if approached cooperatively and given education about hyperemesis. Being honest about your difficulties while highlighting your dedication and work ethic leads to the best outcomes. ***Do not let HG derail your career.***

Adjusting Work Responsibilities During Episodes

During a severe episode of hyperemesis gravidarum, temporarily adjusting work duties and responsibilities often becomes necessary. Options to explore include:

1. **Working from home:** Telecommuting eliminates the commute and allows you to work from bed on difficult days.

2. **Flexible scheduling:** Adjust your hours to start later or take more frequent breaks on nausea-peak days.

3. **Job sharing or shifting:** Transfer some tasks temporarily to capable colleagues to lighten the load.

4. **Reduced hours:** Cut back to part-time hours during the most difficult stretch of HG rather than resigning fully.

5. **Intermittent leave:** Take a few weeks of sick leave during an episode, then return when symptoms improve.

6. **Extended leave:** If needed for health reasons, consider taking a few months off under STD or FMLA to focus on your health.

7. **Remove triggering tasks:** Get help with assignments that require extensive computer work, reading, or travel.

8. **Limit meetings:** Reduce long meetings that can trigger nausea and fatigue. Opt for quick phone or video conferences.

9. **Adjust communication styles:** Use email, messaging, or phone calls more when feeling too ill to meet face-to-face.

10. **Let others lead:** Delegate leadership roles like running meetings or presenting to team members during rough periods.

11. **Block time for self-care:** Schedule breaks for rest, hydration, and snacks as needed.

12. **Set boundaries:** Make your health a priority, and do not let workplace demands impede necessary care. Say no when needed.

The goal is to strike a sustainable balance between work and hyperemesis care. With creative problem-solving, most moms-to-be can find a modified schedule or responsibilities that allow them to remain productive while receiving needed accommodations. ***Do not struggle alone in silence.***

Maintaining a Healthy Work-life Balance

When battling hyperemesis gravidarum, setting boundaries and maintaining a healthy work-life balance are essential but challenging. Strategies that can help include:

1. **Prioritize self-care:** Listen to your body's limits, and do not push yourself to exhaustion in any area of life. Gentleness and moderation are essential.

2. **Let go of guilt:** Remind yourself that taking sick time or saying no to extra duties does not make you lazy or less dedicated. You are doing what is necessary for your health.

3. **Use stress management skills:** practice mindfulness techniques, self-compassion exercises, and counseling to manage anxieties. Reduce unnecessary stressors.

4. **Recruit help:** Call your support network for help with chores, childcare, and other obligations that sap your energy. Outsource what you can.

5. **Adjust standards:** Perfectionism must go out the window when battling HG. Do what you can reasonably manage and let other things slide.

6. **Take things one day at a time:** Focus on getting through just that day on rough days rather than worrying about long-term plans and obligations.

7. **Capitalize on good days or windows:** When you get an episodic burst of energy, use it to catch up judiciously on crucial work or home projects.

8. **Communicate needs clearly:** Remind bosses and colleagues when you have to decline activities due to hyperemesis care. Say no firmly yet politely.

9. **Set small goals:** Break down big tasks into mini-goals you can tackle in as short increments as health allows. Adjust expectations.

10. **Schedule relaxing activities:** Make sure each week includes something enjoyable like a massage, pedicure, date night, or other breather.

11. **Keep perspective:** Remember, this is just a season. Setting realistic priorities now enables success in all spheres later.

Learning to let go of the need for constant productivity frees up energy for self-care. You can emerge from HG as a healthier and more resilient worker and family member with some adjustments.

Chapter 7

Celebrating Small Wins: Success Stories

Inspirational Stories of Overcoming Challenges

Battling hyperemesis gravidarum feels like an endless fight. Drawing inspiration from other women's success stories and concentrating on small daily victories can help you stay motivated.

Maggie constantly vomited up the anti-nausea medications before they could start working. The turning point came when her doctor prescribed a sustained-release pill formulation that finally relieved her symptoms after weeks of struggle.

Cynthia felt crushed and panicked when she was told she would likely need a feeding tube. However, the tube gave her the first full night of sleep and essential nutrition in months. She went on to deliver a healthy baby boy.

Meredith asked her employer to reduce her hours from 40 to 30 weekly. Though it meant some financial sacrifice, the extra time to rest and hydrate allowed her to maintain her job.

Joanna's marriage was strained to the brink by the stress of HG. Seeking couples counseling gave them tools to communicate compassionately and rebuild intimacy after months of hardship.

Sonia's friends did not understand why she kept canceling plans until she helped them read up on HG. Once educated, they stepped up to bring her meals, visit her, and support her mental health.

Casey was bedridden 23 hours a day and rarely showered. When her sister arrived and helped with bathing and skin care, she finally started feeling human again.

Stephanie was sure she would be stuck battling HG for the rest of her pregnancy. Nevertheless, surprisingly, her symptoms started improving at 18 weeks, just as her providers predicted.

Laura was told that pregnancy may exacerbate her chronic migraines. However, implementing headache prevention techniques led to less pain and disability than before pregnancy.

HG makes even simple tasks seem monumental. However, by breaking challenges down into small, daily victories—keeping down the medicine, getting hydrated, making it to appointments—you build the strength to keep marching forward. *You've got this!*

Triumphs in Managing Hyperemesis Gravidarum

Coping with hyperemesis gravidarum often feels like an uphill battle. However, celebrating the daily triumphs along the way, no matter how small, generates hope and momentum. Examples of victories worth relishing include:

- Making it through a work call without having to vomit
- Keeping down prenatal vitamins for a whole week

- Not having to go to the ER for IV fluids for an entire month
- Taking a short walk around the block after weeks in bed
- Managing to eat one balanced meal a day instead of pure carbs
- Seeing your baby move around on an ultrasound, despite the HG battle
- Having the energy to cuddle or read to your older kids
- Going an entire night without waking up to vomit
- Seeing the scale start to stabilize instead of having a downward trend
- Receiving helpful medical advice from a new maternal-fetal medicine specialist
- Finding an anti-nausea medicine that finally provides some relief
- Making it to a close friend's baby shower, even if only briefly
- Having your partner take over chores so you can rest more
- Figuring out which cold foods help settle your stomach

- Seeing supportive social media posts from people cheering you on
- Feeling mentally stronger and less depressed after starting therapy

When every smell, taste, and movement can trigger more vomiting, simply getting through a day without going to urgent care feels like a miracle. Celebrate every positive milestone, therapy success, act of comfort from loved ones, and minor symptom improvement. They will carry you through this season of sickness to the joys ahead. ***You've got this, warrior!***

Community Support and Shared Victories

Battling hyperemesis gravidarum can feel lonely and isolating. Connecting with a community of women fighting the same battle provides solidarity and multiplied strength. Together, you can celebrate shared victories.

Finding an online or in-person HG support group leads to a sense of *"I am not alone in this."* Group members can relate to your daily struggles in a way that even loved ones cannot. Sharing tips on managing work, nausea remedies, finding HG-knowledgeable providers, and safe medications creates a wealth of collective wisdom.

Knowing other women have walked this difficult path and gone on to have healthy babies and families gives hope on dark days when HG feels endless. Their triumphs and postpartum success stories become your inspiration.

Seeing fellow group members cheer you on through setbacks like hospitalizations or feeding tubes makes the process less scary and embarrassing. Their support keeps you fighting.

Groups celebrating the little victories together—making it to your due date, getting diagnosed early, finding an anti-nausea medicine that works—remind you that each small step forward matters.

Having a circle that acknowledges how excruciating HG can be prevents you from feeling like you are exaggerating or *"just complaining."* Their validation helps you feel understood, and their voice struggles freely.

Laughing together about the grossness of vomit bags and burp cloths or how you dream about the foods you will devour postpartum brings some lightness amid the misery.

Sharing about partners, families, or coworkers who finally *"got it"* and stepped up their support makes your burden feel lighter. Their breakthroughs inspire you not to give up on unsupportive loved ones.

Seeing former HG comrades heal and thrive years later with their families depicts the joy ahead. You can get through this season. With communal support, empathy, and wisdom, you withstand the storm. Side-by-side, HG feels like a challenge to overcome, not a hopeless defeat. ***You've got this, mama!***

Chapter 8

Planning for the Future: Family and Beyond

Family Planning Considerations after Hyperemesis Gravidarum

For women who endure hyperemesis gravidarum, contemplating future pregnancies can elicit a mix of emotions. Navigating family planning decisions in light of HG requires thoughtfulness and open conversations.

It is normal to feel torn between longing for more children and fear of reliving HG's trauma. Up to 80% of HG pregnancies result in recurrence, but severity varies. Understanding your priorities and risks is key.

If you hope to expand your family, preconception counseling provides a chance to develop a proactive HG management plan. Testing for conditions like thyroid disease, discussing genetic factors, and adjusting medications and supplements pre-pregnancy may help. Being closely monitored from the start and considering IV hydration from weeks 4-5 onward can lessen the severity for some.

For others, the physical and emotional toll may preclude further biological children. Evaluating options like surrogacy and adoption as alternate paths can aid the grieving process. Accepting that "your family is complete" despite your desires takes courage.

If you are considering permanent contraception, give yourself ample time and counseling support to process complex emotions. Tubal ligation in the fog of HG recovery can elicit regret. Pausing to let the intensity subside enables wise decisions.

Open communication, self-compassion, and hope are critical in any circumstance. You are more than HG; let its shadow shrink, not darken your horizon. Try visualizing future joy.

Your provider, counselor, and support network offer wisdom and comfort in weighing options. Ultimately, listen to your heart; this journey has many correct answers. You can craft a beautiful life however you choose. Healing is possible.

Pregnancy Outlook for Subsequent Pregnancies

For women who experienced hyperemesis gravidarum (HG) in a previous pregnancy, wondering if future conceptions will mean battling HG again is common. While there are no guarantees, these fundamental facts help set realistic expectations:

- **The recurrence risk is high but not certain.** Around 80% of women with prior HG experience it in later pregnancies. However, 20% do not, so hope remains.
- **Severity varies.** Subsequent HG can be similar, milder, or more severe than past episodes. Unpredictability causes uncertainty.
- **The risk increases with multiple prior HG pregnancies.** Women who endure HG through two or more pregnancies have 95% or higher recurrence odds.

- **HG peaks in weeks 8–12 and then often improves.** Later pregnancies may mirror or extend this pattern.
- **Medications and IV hydration can temper the severity.** Implementing interventions proactively may circumvent complications.
- **Each pregnancy differs.** Unique circumstances like age, weight changes, or shifting life stresses can affect susceptibility.
- **Genetics underlie recurrence.** The family history of HG hints at future risk.
- **Providers grow more proficient.** Their experience with your history can lead to better management.

While the odds of battling HG again may seem daunting, physicians emphasize that the prognosis remains hopeful. Having a knowledgeable care team monitor you closely enables early detection and rapid treatment if nausea and vomiting recur.

Understanding triggers and effective interventions from past pregnancies equips you to advocate for appropriate care quickly. Entering a subsequent pregnancy educated and proactive is key. Seeking counseling to process complex emotions also helps smooth the journey.

Your needs come first; be empowered to make family planning choices that align with your priorities and values. With support, compassion, and hope, you can successfully navigate whatever course lies ahead.

Long-term Effects and Postpartum Recovery

In the throes of unrelenting nausea and vomiting, coping day-to-day with hyperemesis gravidarum often consumes all energy and thought. However, understanding the long-term effects and postpartum recovery course can help you look beyond the present darkness.

The good news is that, in most cases, HG symptoms begin to resolve and disappear entirely for the majority of women by delivery or soon after. Your body and mind start healing. However, study data reveals that anywhere from 25–50% of HG survivors continue to battle residual effects postpartum.

- Persistent anxiety or depression
- Post-traumatic stress-type symptoms
- Eating disorders or food aversions that developed during HG
- Neurological effects like memory problems

- Loss of muscle tone and lingering fatigue or weakness
- Continued gastrointestinal issues like reflux
- Kidney problems from recurrent dehydration
- Lingering vitamin and mineral deficiencies
- Relationship strain that arose during the HG period

Seeking supportive mental health services, proper nutrition, physical/pelvic floor therapy, and compassionate caregivers optimizes recovery. Give yourself ample time to regain strength holistically.

While shadows of HG may remain for some, many women find their joy and zest for life blossoming again without constant nausea and vomiting. Your body remembers wellness and newfound gratitude emerges.

Focus on HG is a season, not your forever fate. Let go of guilt, perfectionism, and the need to "bounce back" overnight. Healing takes time, so be gentle with yourself. ***The light ahead awaits.***

Chapter 9

Advocacy and Awareness

Promoting Awareness about Hyperemesis Gravidarum

Despite its potentially severe impact on maternal and fetal health, public awareness of hyperemesis gravidarum (HG) remains limited. By speaking out and sharing your story, you can raise consciousness to help other women get diagnosed and treated promptly. Ways to promote HG awareness include:

- **Educating loved ones.** Ensure your friends, family, and partner understand this is a real medical condition, not just bad morning sickness. Share HG facts and stories to foster empathy.

- **Contacting local media.** Pitch your story to local news and radio outlets to communicate the serious need for HG awareness and treatment improvements.

- **Speaking at public events.** Look for opportunities to present your experience at community forums focused on women's health and family issues.

- **Working with non-profits.** Partner with organizations like the HER Foundation to participate in fundraising and awareness campaigns.

- **Joining patient advocacy groups.** Add your voice to national groups like the Hyperemesis Education and Research (HER) Foundation that lobby and educate on behalf of HG patients.

- **Attending rallies/conferences.** Look for local and national events bringing the HG community together to be further empowered.

- **Writing op-eds or blogs.** Share your challenges and triumphs in a blog for a parenting website or submit an editorial to news outlets.

- **Creating informational displays.** Design exhibits about HG to be displayed at libraries, clinics, and community centers (especially during pregnancy awareness month).

- **Contacting legislators.** Communicate the need for better HG education and treatment to your state and federally elected officials.
- **Sharing in support groups.** Take your HG support group lessons to your social networks to elevate understanding.
- **Posting on social media.** Use personal accounts and hashtags like #HyperemesisGravidarum and #HGAwareness to share facts and stories.

Every woman battling HG who speaks up makes a difference. We can educate providers, policymakers, and the public to transform misperceptions about "morning sickness." Break the isolation and shame by boldly sharing your experience. ***You are a warrior!***

Advocacy Efforts for Improved Medical Understanding

While awareness of hyperemesis gravidarum is gradually increasing, continued advocacy efforts focused on improving medical providers' understanding and approach to this condition remain critical to ensuring women promptly get the treatment they need.

Key ways to advocate for better provider education include:

- **Bringing fact sheets and research to appointments.** Share current literature on HG risks, diagnosis, and management with your OB and nurses. Educate them gently.

- **Ask about their HG experience or training.** Understand their background in recognizing and treating severe nausea or vomiting during pregnancy. Choose specialists wisely.

- **Provide feedback.** If you feel your concerns have been minimized or proper treatment delayed, tactfully relay that so they can improve. File formal complaints only if needed.

- **Connect providers to resources.** Point them to informative sites like HelpHer.org and suggest HG-focused webinars or conferences.

- **Ask for explanations.** When guidance seems misguided or dismissive, ask clarifying questions to illuminate flawed thinking and assumptions.

- **Request consultation referrals.** If your current team needs HG management expertise, push for a perinatal medicine specialist to consult.

- **Share your complete history.** Fully communicating symptoms, weight loss patterns, and prior treatments helps them appropriately evaluate severity and progression.

- **Lobbying physician organizations.** Work with groups like the HER Foundation to better integrate HG education into OBGYN training and CPD courses.

- **Advocate for research.** Support initiatives to expand HG-focused research to clarify optimal diagnostic and treatment protocols based on evidence.

- **Join hospital advisory boards.** Having an HG patient perspective represented when developing women's health programming helps reshape institutional culture.

- **Petition insurance companies.** Push for HG treatments and extended hospitalizations to be adequately covered and deemed medically necessary.

By persistently yet professionally urging those in power to understand this underrecognized condition better, you create positive ripples for women facing HG now and in the future. ***Your efforts pave the way.***

Support Organizations and Resources

When struggling with hyperemesis gravidarum, connecting to organizations and accessing resources created by women who have walked in your shoes provides invaluable information and support. Key groups include:

- **HER Foundation:** HER stands for "Hyperemesis Education and Research." This non-profit was founded in 2010 to provide patient support and advocate for HG education. It has local chapters and fundraises for HG research and provider training. Their website contains webinars, research, articles, and more.
www.HelpHER.org

- **The HER HG Community on Facebook:** This is a giant online support group community moderated by HER Foundation volunteers. Over 14,000 members share guidance, hope, and understanding. Women connect and build each other up.

- **International Kates Club for Hyperemesis Gravidarum:** Named after a woman who suffered from HG, this group provides a forum to share treatment reviews, coping tips, provider recommendations, and emotional support. **www.katesclub.org**

- **Hyperemesis Research:** A UK-based organization funding studies and clinical trials on HG prevention, treatment, and care. Their research helps expand medical understanding and care worldwide. **www.hyperemesis.org.uk**

- **Hyperemesis UK:** Provides education and support services to empower women with HG in the United Kingdom. They have downloadable hospital care plans that women can share with their providers. **www.PregnancySicknessSupport.org.uk**

- **HER HG Pregnancy app:** Helps women track symptoms, hydration, weight loss, and interventions. Save records easily to share with your providers. Connects you to HER resources and community. **BecomingHER app**

These organizations shine a light in the darkness of HG. By taking advantage of their resources, patient advocacy power multiplies. You gain knowledge, hope, and sisterhood.

Chapter 10

Addressing Myths and Stigmas

Common Myths Surrounding Morning Sickness

Hyperemesis gravidarum is already highly misunderstood. On top of that, various myths and misconceptions about general pregnancy nausea and "morning sickness" further complicate efforts to improve awareness and treatment. Common morning sickness myths include:

Myth: *By the beginning of the second trimester, morning sickness usually goes away.*

Fact: For most women, it improves, but up to 20% continue battling nausea and vomiting past week 14.

Myth: Morning sickness is caused by hormonal changes and indicates a healthy pregnancy.

Fact: While hCG does play a role, severe nausea and vomiting are never normal or healthy.

Myth: Eating crackers the first thing in the morning prevents nausea.

Fact: No food can prevent morning sickness, though some women report that this strategy temporarily relieves mild queasiness.

Myth: Morning sickness that requires medications means a "high-needs pregnancy."

Fact: Seeking medical relief for a legitimate health condition makes you an empowered patient, not someone with "high needs."

Myth: Ginger ale and sea bands cure morning sickness.

Fact: Some women get mild relief from alternative remedies, but most require standard antiemetic medications.

Myth: Pregnancy nausea is just an inconvenience women must power through.

Fact: Nausea and vomiting during pregnancy can have significant adverse health impacts if not properly treated.

Myth: *Morning sickness impacts all pregnant women the same.*

Fact: Symptom severity varies greatly based on multiple factors. HG is not just a standard morning sickness that intensifies.

The key is distinguishing fact from fiction when it comes to general nausea versus severe vomiting during pregnancy. Educating loved ones to ignore myths helps them understand that your HG battle is real and serious. Facts fight stigma.

Breaking Down Stigmas Associated with Hyperemesis Gravidarum

Far too often, the severe nausea and vomiting of hyperemesis gravidarum get minimized as "just a normal part of pregnancy." This contributes to women being discriminated against, judged, and denied needed accommodations. Breaking the dangerous stigma around HG is imperative. Common problematic attitudes toward HG that propagate stigma include:

- Viewing HG as an exaggeration or overreaction to regular pregnancy nausea
- Assuming women bring it upon themselves through anxiety or poor self-care
- Judging women as 'weak' or complainers for struggling to work through it
- Blaming women for using HG as an 'excuse' to shirk responsibilities
- Pressuring women to 'power through' the symptoms without accommodations
- Discrediting HG as a real medical condition requiring intensive treatment
- Criticizing women for seeking medication instead of 'going natural'
- Minimizing the impact of HG on women's health and families
- Recommending unproven folk remedies while ignoring medical advice
- Discouraging women from getting feeding tubes by emphasizing cosmetic effects

Changing these damaging mindsets begins with sharing facts that counter misinformation. HG is a legitimate diagnosis with severe risks requiring medical intervention, not a choice or personal failure. Appropriate accommodations allow women to maintain families and careers safely for the long term. Support enables thriving.

Every woman who bravely shares their story publicly dismantles shame and stigma. We must speak up and say hyperemesis gravidarum's toll is real. Our community deserves compassion, not judgment or dismissal. Together, we can transform understanding worldwide.

Educating the Society for a More Supportive Environment

A critical step in de-stigmatizing hyperemesis gravidarum involves broadly educating all levels of society about its reality and severe effects. Increased public awareness creates a more supportive environment for the HG community.

Strategies for effectively educating society include the following:

- Share personal stories and HG facts through the media. Getting HG featured in large publications, TV outlets, and social media expands general understanding.
- Distribute literature to clinics and pregnancy organizations. Ensure brochures and flyers

illuminating HG are available at OBGYN offices, birthing centers, midwife groups, and women's organizations.

- Speak at high schools and universities. Lecturing about your experience with HG in health classes and on college campuses spreads awareness to younger generations.

- Advocate for coverage in prenatal classes. Request that HG symptoms, risks, and treatment be integrated into standard childbirth preparation courses' curriculums.

- Train supportive nurses and doulas. Ensure care professionals interacting closely with pregnant women receive proper education about recognizing and compassionately responding to HG.

- Create awareness months and events. Getting HG highlighted annually during critical months like September for Pregnancy Sickness Awareness Month reinforces public attention.

- Lobby policymakers. Push legislators to increase funding for HG research and treatment access to bring about change on a systemic level.

- Partner with private companies. Collaborate with businesses that serve expectant mothers, like maternity clothing brands, to integrate HG education into their platforms.

Broadening HG's understanding transforms workplaces, clinical settings, friend circles, families, and public venues into more supportive spaces for the warriors battling this problematic condition. You deserve love, not judgment. ***Together, we build change.***

Chapter 11

Expert Insights: Interviews and Professional Opinions

Conversations with Healthcare Professionals

Gaining insights from physicians, nurses, and other experts caring for hyperemesis gravidarum patients provides invaluable perspectives. Their experience illuminates practical guidance and compassion.

In an interview, **Dr. Samuel, a high-risk OBGYN, shares:** *"I never downplay how miserable and isolating HG can feel during pregnancy. But I remind patients that the storm will pass with proper treatment and support, and they will* *get their lives back. Catching it early and controlling symptoms is key."*

Nurse Theresa emphasizes:

"Women with HG need our empathy as much as medical care. I let them know that their struggles are real and valid. Our job is to support them both physically and emotionally through this tough season."

Dietitian Lauren adds:

"The focus cannot be on 'fixing' the diet to stop HG but rather finding any nutrients that a woman can tolerate and keep down. Small, frequent meals with hydrating fluids usually work best when battling constant nausea."

Acupuncturist Marissa shares:

"While acupuncture alone won't cure hyperemesis gravidarum, my patients say it provides welcome relief between medications and IV treatments. I aim to reduce their discomfort and anxiety levels."

These knowledgeable specialists provide tips and reveal compassion. Seeking multidisciplinary input aids in treatment and recovery.

Insights from Nutritionists and Mental Health Experts

In addition to maternal-fetal medicine doctors, obstetricians, and nurses, experts like dietitians, social workers, and therapists offer invaluable guidance for effectively managing hyperemesis gravidarum.

Nutritionist Samantha explains:

"The priority with HG is getting any calories and hydration in versus sticking to a 'perfect' diet. Small nibbles of crackers, popsicles, ginger ale—whatever stays down and provides fuel during relentless nausea."

Registered dietitian Amanda notes:

"I work with women to determine beverages, foods, vitamins, and menus that trigger less nausea. Boost shakes or liquid nutrition may be needed if weight loss exceeds 10%."

Therapist Dana shares:

"It's understandable for HG moms to feel resentful, depressed, and guilty. My role is to validate those feelings and teach coping skills to nurture mental health amid the suffering."

Social worker Lauren adds:

"In addition to medical care, connecting women to local support groups, counseling services, respite childcare, and workplace accommodations improves quality of life and relationships."

Leveraging expertise across specialties ensures that physical and emotional needs are supported through challenging HG pregnancies. Seeking diverse perspectives leads to more holistic care.

Research Findings and Ongoing Studies

While hyperemesis gravidarum remains under-researched compared to many conditions, insightful studies examining prevalence, risk factors, treatments, and impacts continue to expand medical understanding.

Recent research findings include:

- HG impacts up to 3% of pregnancies in the US, causing over 250,000 ER visits annually.
- Women hospitalized for HG have a 3.6-fold increased risk of preterm birth.
- Genetic mutations related to vitamin A and iron metabolism may underlie HG susceptibility.

- Women with anxiety disorders have 85% higher odds of experiencing HG symptoms.
- Ondansetron is the most widely studied and utilized HG antiemetic medication, with relatively low fetal risks.
- Weekly outpatient IV fluid therapy reduces HG hospitalization rates by 60% compared to oral hydration alone.
- Women rank the most helpful components of HG care as IV fluids, antiemetics, enteral nutrition, and psychoemotional support.

Ongoing studies aim to:

- Uncover prognostic biomarkers to predict HG severity and guide treatment plans.
- Develop new pharmaceutical interventions that effectively curb nausea while minimizing fetal exposure.
- Optimize nutritional support protocols at home and in clinical settings.
- Clarify the safety profiles and dosage guidelines for existing antiemetic medications.
- Reduce the workplace stigma and socioeconomic burdens experienced by women disabled by HG.

While gaps remain in fully understanding and managing HG, researchers make promising strides each year thanks to funding and volunteers. Their breakthroughs pave the way for improved diagnosis, treatment, and support.

Chapter 12

Personal Growth and Resilience

Building Resilience Through Adversity

Though the physical and emotional tolls of hyperemesis gravidarum often feel crushingly heavy at the moment, looking back, many women describe emerging from the battle with newfound resilience, perspective, and strength.

Fighting through HG builds resilience in powerful ways:

1. **Physical toughness:** Your body learns it can survive and heal from depletions it once thought would break you.

2. **Resourcefulness:** You determine how to function and meet needs despite unrelenting obstacles.

3. **Self-advocacy:** You find your voice to stand up for your health needs against dismissing systems.

4. **Help-seeking:** You shed pride and ask for assistance, realizing you do not need to do life alone.

5. **Adaptability:** Adjusting plans while mourning lost dreams helps you flex to meet new realities.

6. **Gratitude:** Suffering teaches you not to take simple joys like food, activity, and comfort for granted.

7. **Presence:** HG forces you to focus on getting through each day and living more presently.

8. **Self-compassion:** You stop judging yourself and embrace imperfection and gentleness.

9. **Perspective:** What once seemed huge pales when compared to the challenges you have endured.

10. **Empathy:** You better understand the pain of others battling chronic illness or disability.

11. **Wisdom:** You gain tools and knowledge to pass on to other women facing HG in the future.

While it takes time to recognize the silver linings, know that your capacity to handle hardship has expanded. You are stronger for having survived the storm.

Discovering Strength in Challenging Moments

When immersed in nonstop nausea, vomiting, and disability, mustering any sense of inner strength can seem impossible for women battling hyperemesis gravidarum. However, even on the darkest days, we can find reserves of courage and resilience we never knew existed.

Moments that reveal unexpected strength include:

- Asking for IV fluids again despite the embarrassment of repeated ER trips
- Reaching out to friends even when you feel too sick to socialize at all
- Letting other moms see your feeding tube and sharing tips to help them
- Opening up about depression instead of continuing to struggle silently
- Switching doctors when you need better care, despite loyalty pressures
- Sharing an unfiltered photo of your HG pregnancy weight loss and bloat
- Leaving a partner unwilling to support you through HG despite financial fears
- Returning to work part-time earlier than planned to maintain normalcy

- Advocating firmly for accommodations from unsupportive bosses
- Sharing your story publicly to combat stigma despite humiliation
- Deciding your family is complete despite the pressure to have "just one more."
- Asking relatives to take the kids for a weekend when you desperately need rest
- Choosing to end a pregnancy that is exacerbating your health risks

Though each situation differs, we consistently discover wells of grit that deepen our courage and capabilities. HG proves you are stronger than you know.

Lessons Learned from My Journey

As I reflect on my personal hyperemesis gravidarum journey, that difficult season taught me invaluable life lessons that forever changed me for the better.

I learned:

1. **How strong I can be:** I survived challenges I never dreamed possible. This fortified my confidence in handling future trials.

2. **To let go of control:** HG showed me I cannot control everything. I practiced accepting help and surrendering to limits.

3. **The art of adapting:** With plans derailed by HG, I discovered how to pivot and modify expectations flexibly.

4. **Who my faithful supporters are:** I am now more intentional about nurturing relationships that brought me comfort during the depths.

5. **Not to judge others' pain:** Witnessing the concern in my husband's eyes taught me to empathize better with those hurting.

6. **How blessed I am:** HG gave me renewed gratitude for the basic gifts of health, mobility, and comfort I had taken for granted.

7. **Nutrition matters:** I gained an appreciation for my body's needs and fuel after malnutrition took its toll.

8. **To use my voice:** Advocating for my care against dismissive doctors empowered me to speak up in all areas.

9. **Rest is productive:** HG required learning to relinquish guilt over "unproductive" time spent simply healing.

10. **Progress happens slowly:** Just as HG subsided gradually, so do most life changes requiring patience.

11. **Hope sustains:** When I despaired of HG lasting forever, digging into stories of others recovering after delivery encouraged me.

HG asked everything of me, both physically and mentally. Rising to its challenges expanded my skills, priorities, compassion, and worldview. I emerged mightier for having survived the crucible.

Chapter 13

The Role of Partners and Loved Ones

Supporting a Partner with Hyperemesis Gravidarum

Caring for a partner battling hyperemesis gravidarum brings unique challenges. However, you play a critical role in helping her cope. With understanding and proactive support, you can ease her struggle.

Important ways partners can help include:

1. **Educating yourself:** Learn all you can about HG symptoms, treatments, and impacts to understand her challenges.

2. **Encouraging medical care:** Help her get IV fluids, medications, and nutrition support on difficult days. Drive her to appointments.

3. **Communicating:** Ask how she feels and listen without trying to "fix" it. Validate her emotions.

4. **Helping around the home:** Take on cooking, cleaning, errands, and childcare duties if needed. Do not wait to be asked.

5. **Offering respite:** Give her time to rest away from demands and noise. Create a comfortable sanctuary.

6. **Providing comfort:** Bring items to ease her discomfort, like popsicles, tea, cold washcloths, and lip balm.

7. **Finding solutions together:** When tensions rise, avoid blaming and gently brainstorm compromises.

8. **Sharing feelings:** Open up when you feel scared, overwhelmed, or neglected without making her responsible.

9. **Being affectionate:** Offer hugs, handholding, and other intimacy that nourish the relationship.

10. **Celebrating milestones:** Note that each day, she makes it through, has weight regained, and has a good test result.

With a compassionate, partnered approach, you build each other up. Your devotion and sacrifice during her HG battle will reap dividends, strengthening your lifelong bond.

Involving Family and Friends in the Journey

Hyperemesis gravidarum can feel extremely isolating, but inviting loved ones into your struggle appropriately provides invaluable emotional and practical support.

Ways to thoughtfully involve family and friends:

1. **Educate about HG.** Share articles and resources so they understand this diagnosis goes beyond morning sickness. Correct misperceptions.

2. **Be specific about your needs.** Give clear ideas of how they can tangibly help, like meals, rides to appointments, or childcare, rather than just asking, "Let me know if I can help."

3. **Communicate limitations.** Explain your low stamina so they do not feel hurt if you decline visits, baby showers, or parties.

4. **Allow help.** Accept offers of support even when they go against inclinations toward independence and privacy.

5. **Provide new ways to connect.** If you are up for brief texting or front porch visits, invite them instead of doing nothing.

6. **Share your heart.** Being open about fears, frustrations, and needs for encouragement invites greater intimacy. Let them carry this burden with you.

7. **Give reassurance.** When you decline invitations, emphasize that they are temporary for this season and that you still love them.

8. **Normalize messiness.** Let friends see your sickness and house chaos without pressure to constantly put on a happy face.

9. **Discuss birth plans.** Involve them in conversations about your ideal delivery experience and postpartum help.

10. **Express gratitude.** Send thank-you notes or texts to acknowledge acts of service and friendship that uplift you.

While setting needed boundaries, let loved ones fully into your HG experience. Their support lightens the challenges and deepens your connections.

Strengthening Relationships through Shared Experiences

At times, hyperemesis gravidarum can strain relationships as loved ones struggle to relate and tensions mount. However, even amid hardship, inviting others into your experience in positive ways often deepens bonds and fortifies love.

You strengthen ties when you:

1. **Share ultrasound images.** Even when feeling sick, include them in your baby's development.
2. **Let them bring you comfort.** Their acts of service and care for you convey love.
3. **Educate them.** Explaining HG facts helps garner empathy and dispel misperceptions straining the relationship.
4. **Cry together.** Being vulnerable to fear and pain fosters intimacy.
5. **Reassure them.** Alleviate unwarranted guilt by conveying your confidence in their support.
6. **Involve them in appointments.** Having your partner, mom, or friend come to crucial doctor visits helps them grasp the medical realities you are facing.

7. **Ask for their opinions.** Getting their input on big decisions honors their care for you.

8. **Foster openness.** Avoid masking struggles and instead unveil your authentic journey, inviting uncomplicated support.

9. **Share your wins.** Expressing excitement over even minor symptom improvements and milestones allows them to celebrate along your road to better health.

10. **Look to the future.** Discuss your hopes about your growing family, relationship dreams, and plans post-HG.

11. **Show gratitude.** Frequently thank them for walking this challenging road with you and acknowledge acts of sacrifice.

While HG adds a unique strain, seeing loved ones rise to the challenges with devotion often ignites newfound joy, respect, and unity. You do not have to walk alone. Together, you will make it through the storm.

Chapter 14

Future Perspectives: Medical Advances and Research

Ongoing Research for Hyperemesis Gravidarum

While hyperemesis gravidarum remains less studied than many pregnancy complications, dedicated researchers make meaningful strides each year in better understanding and treating this difficult condition through scientific studies.

Key areas of focus include:

1. **Genetic underpinnings:** Scientists work to identify specific gene variants that influence HG

susceptibility and severity. This allows for better risk assessment.

2. **Biomarker discovery:** Distinct compounds in blood or urine that reliably predict and track HG could enable earlier diagnosis and interventions.

3. **Improved medications:** A priority is developing more effective anti-nausea drugs that minimize fetal exposure or defects risks.

4. **Alternative therapies:** Smaller studies explore acupuncture, acupressure, vitamin B6, ginger, magnesium, and more for reducing symptoms.

5. **Optimized nutrition:** Researchers examine formulas and protocols to most effectively provide hydration and sustain maternal and fetal nutrition in HG.

6. **Mental health impact:** Experts further evaluate depression, anxiety, PTSD, and quality of life experiences among HG patients to improve psychosocial care.

7. **Health economics:** Analyzing the total costs of hospitalizations, lost work productivity, and other burdens quantifies HG's societal impact and need for solutions.

8. **Provider education:** Surveys and focus groups assess gaps in medical teams' knowledge of HG to shape better curriculum and training.

Each study brings us one step closer to the day when more women are quickly diagnosed, new medications curb symptoms, stigma fades, and full support is readily accessible. ***The future is full of hope.***

Potential Breakthroughs in Treatment

As hyperemesis gravidarum research steadily expands scientific understanding of its causes and impacts, experts anticipate vital breakthroughs that promise to transform prevention and treatment in the coming decade.

Future advances may include:

1. **A prognostic genetic panel:** A lab test identifying women with gene variants putting them at high HG risk could enable preventative steps pre-pregnancy.

2. **Biomarker screening:** Checking levels of certain compounds could provide an early HG diagnosis and indicate severity to customize care.

3. **New antiemetic drugs:** Pharmaceuticals currently in development may better control nausea with fewer fetal side effects and maternal health risks.

4. **Targeted vitamins and nutrients:** Tailored IV supplementation based on individual deficiencies found through testing may improve maternal outcomes.

5. **Gut microbiome modulation:** Altering gut bacteria composition through diet, probiotics, or fecal transplants may influence HG susceptibility and inflammation, driving nausea.

6. **Acupuncture efficacy:** Larger randomized studies may confirm acupuncture's benefits for reducing HG severity and enhancing provider adoption.

7. **Breakthrough dietary formulas:** New medical food products and formulas may better sustain hydration and nutrition in severe cases.

8. **Expanded patient registries:** Large databases tracking women throughout pregnancy will reveal long-term insights and enable big data analytics.

9. **Artificial intelligence risk calculators:** Complex algorithms could help predict prognosis, guide treatment plans, and monitor patients remotely using data like symptoms, genetics, and biomarkers.

While HG remains challenging to prevent, experts foresee many avenues for reducing suffering and complications through earlier diagnosis and improved, personalized interventions. ***Exciting progress lies ahead!***

Hope for a Brighter Future

When caught in relentless cycles of nausea, vomiting, and disability, hyperemesis can feel like it will never end and diminish all joy in pregnancy. However, as research steadily progresses and care improves, there is tremendous hope for a brighter future for HG moms-to-be. Reasons to be optimistic include:

1. **Increased awareness and validation:** Today's mothers no longer need to suffer silently without answers, thanks to the growing public consciousness of HG's severity.

2. **Earlier diagnosis:** With improved provider education and awareness among women, HG is detected earlier, allowing treatment to begin as soon as possible.

3. **Support networks:** Online groups and nonprofits help women feel less alone and more empowered to advocate for their needs. Help is out there.

4. **Medication improvements:** Though imperfect, new drugs help control nausea better with fewer risks than options decades ago.

5. **IV therapy advancements:** Greater access to at-home and outpatient infusion keeps more women from requiring hospitalization.

6. **Nutritional formulas:** Products like tube feeding, shakes, and IV vitamin cocktails prevent dangerous malnutrition.

7. **Work policy evolution:** Updated pregnancy disability laws and remote work options provide needed job flexibility for HG patients.

8. **Mental health integration:** Counseling and support groups now address HG's emotional aspects and physical needs.

9. **Scientific momentum:** Research studies steadily drive the discovery of new treatments and approaches to managing symptoms.

10. **Hopeful stories:** Other women who have survived HG and gone on to have healthy families show that this season will pass. The light shines ahead.

While HG's hardship remains real today, concentrating on the meaningful progress underway breeds a sense of optimistic anticipation. Your struggle is paving the way for better care for future mothers.

Conclusion

As you approach the end of your hyperemesis gravidarum journey and the delivery of your baby draws near, taking time to reflect on the transformative experience can bring healing and perspective.

Look back with gentleness on:

1. **Your incredible strength:** You survived challenges no one should face, yet you persisted. Honor your grit.

2. **Supports that uplifted:** Appreciate loved ones and providers who cared for you through huge acts or simple gestures.

3. **Skills gained:** You have learned much from advocacy, coping strategies, and medical knowledge. These tools equip your future.

4. **Growth through grief:** Allow yourself to grieve dreams lost or deferred by HG while embracing the personal expansion hardship can bring.

5. **Moments of joy:** Cherish milestones like seeing your baby's face on the ultrasound or feeling their first kick, even if fleeting.

6. **A fuller life view:** HG gave you renewed gratitude for health, deepened empathy for others in pain, and clarified your priorities.

7. **Hope is renewed:** As symptoms subside, optimism emerges. This, too, shall pass.

8. **Love revealed:** The devotion of your partner through the darkness, fatigue, fear, and strain defines real commitment.

9. **A mother's heart:** You carried and protected a new life despite relentless challenges. You gave it all.

As this poignant chapter of profound purpose closes, look ahead with expectancy. Your precious baby will soon make its way into your loving arms. A journey of resilience lies behind you. A bright new horizon awaits.

A Recap on Key Strategies for Survival

As you navigate the daily struggles of hyperemesis gravidarum, remembering these key strategies and coping tips can help empower you to survive each difficult day:

- **Ask for help.** Do not struggle alone. Reach out to loved ones, hire help, and take others up on support offers.

- **Stay hydrated.** Sip fluids all day long and get IV hydration if needed to prevent dangerous dehydration.

- **Take medications.** Use prescribed anti-nausea and acid-reducing medications to control vomiting. Communicate with your provider if they are not effective.

- **Rest and conserve energy.** Getting adequate sleep, taking sick days, and limiting activities prevent exhaustion.

- **Identify safe foods.** Stick to bland, easy-to-digest foods that you can keep down, like toast, rice, potatoes, oatmeal, and applesauce.

- **Get counseling.** Work with a therapist to manage fear, anxiety, depression, and relationship challenges. You do not have to power through this alone.

- **Join a supportive community.** Connect with other HG moms online or locally to combat isolation and get advice.
- **Educate your loved ones.** Share HG facts and stories so friends and family understand your seriousness and support you appropriately.
- **Plan for the hospital.** Pack a bag, arrange childcare, and understand insurance coverage if hospitalization becomes necessary for hydration or nutrition.
- **Celebrate small wins.** Mark any positive step, like making it to work for a few hours or taking a short walk. Give yourself credit for each act of perseverance.

You are strong. You are brave. You are not alone. Take it day by day, hour by hour, if needed. This season will pass. Relief is near. You've got this, mama! We're cheering you on.

Encouraging Others to Share Their Stories

Your personal hyperemesis gravidarum story holds power—the power to help other women feel less alone, gain insights, and resolve to advocate for their care boldly. By courageously sharing your experience, you become part of transforming the HG journey for other families.

Ways to share your story and encourage others include:

1. **Writing compassionately.** Craft a social media post, blog, or article conveying your HG journey. Let your vulnerability and emotions create a connection.

2. **Highlight the highlights.** Reflecting on special moments, like feeling your baby's first kick or admiring their ultrasound photo, counters the narrative of only darkness and despair.

3. **Get specific.** Details about symptoms, effective medications, or nutrition tips can directly help another reader.

4. **Note the support that lifted you.** Give shoutouts to providers, relatives, friends, or partners who made a difference so others know care exists.

5. **Share diverse perspectives.** Unique voices like women of color, single moms, LGBTQ+, low-income, or disabled moms showcase the breadth of HG's reach.

6. **Frame HG as a season.** Remind readers that this difficult chapter will pass, not define their whole life. There is hope ahead.

7. **Celebrate recovery and growth.** The moments you regained strength or perspective demonstrate life beyond hyperemesis.

8. **Highlight advocacy resources.** Share organizations like the HER Foundation that offer education, connection, and empowerment.

9. **Convey courage over perfection.** Admitting challenging moments allows others to voice their struggles without shame.

Your story forges understanding and reform by unveiling the whole patient experience in all its humanity. You never walk alone when generations of women lock arms through shared stories of resilience.

A Message of Hope for Those Battling Hyperemesis Gravidarum

If you are reading this while in the throes of hyperemesis gravidarum's relentless nausea, vomiting, and devastation, please know that this season of suffering will pass. Brighter days will come again. Hope lives.

I see you, brave warrior. I know the agonizing battle you wage each day against your own body to protect the new life within. I know the tears, the pleading prayers, and the crushing isolation. I know it feels endless. Nevertheless, you are so much stronger than this momentary affliction.

Please take comfort in the fact that thousands of people before you have survived this journey and gone on to hold their beautiful, healthy babies in their arms at last. As research progresses, more tools emerge to help mitigate HG's toll.

Though support may seem scarce, there are those ready to lift you: loved ones, doctors, husbands, and friends. Reach out your hand and let them help shoulder your burden. You were meant to walk this road with others.

Celebrate each mini triumph, whether simply keeping down fluids for an hour or making it to an important milestone. Mark each day you move forward. Hold on to stories of hope. When despair surrounds, let stubborn light shine through.

I wonder if HG moms glimpse the true grit of motherhood early—that love often requires everything while giving nothing but reward in return. Take pride in your warrior spirit. You are a powerful mother already.

Soon, this season will fade, but your strength will remain. You will emerge mightier from the crucible. Joy will greet you. Furthermore, we will link arms, a circle of those who have been there, lifting others in their journey too. ***Take heart, momma. You've got this.***

www.ingramcontent.com/pod-product-compliance
Lightning Source LLC
Chambersburg PA
CBHW070859260726
48661CB00004B/1497